Table Of Contents

Chapter 1: Understanding Metabolism

What is metabolism?

In order to achieve lasting weight loss success, it is crucial to understand the concept of metabolism. Metabolism refers to the chemical processes that occur within the body to maintain life. It is responsible for converting food into energy, which fuels all of the body's functions. Essentially, metabolism is the rate at which your body burns calories to maintain vital functions such as breathing, circulation, and digestion. By understanding how metabolism works, you can make lifestyle changes that will rev up your metabolism and promote weight loss.

One natural way to boost metabolism is through regular exercise. Physical activity not only burns calories during the activity itself but also boosts metabolism for hours afterward. Strength training, in particular, can increase muscle mass, which in turn increases the body's resting metabolic rate. This means that even when you are not exercising, your body will be burning more calories. Incorporating a mix of cardiovascular and strength training exercises into your routine can help rev up your metabolism and aid in weight loss.

Metabolism-boosting foods and supplements can also play a role in promoting weight loss. Foods such as lean proteins, whole grains, fruits, and vegetables can help rev up your metabolism by providing essential nutrients that support healthy metabolic function. Additionally, certain supplements like green tea extract, caffeine, and capsaicin have been shown to increase metabolism and promote fat burning. By incorporating these metabolism-boosting foods and supplements into your diet, you can support your body's natural metabolic processes and aid in weight loss.

Making metabolism-boosting lifestyle changes can also have a significant impact on weight loss. Getting an adequate amount of sleep, managing stress levels, and staying hydrated are all important factors in supporting a healthy metabolism. Lack of sleep and high stress levels can disrupt hormonal balance and slow down metabolism, making it harder to lose weight. By prioritizing self-care and adopting healthy habits, you can support your body's metabolic function and make weight loss more achievable.

In conclusion, understanding metabolism is key to achieving lasting weight loss success. By incorporating natural ways to boost metabolism, metabolism-boosting foods and supplements, metabolism-boosting lifestyle changes, and metabolism-boosting tips into your daily routine, you can rev up your metabolism and support your weight loss goals. With a holistic approach to metabolism, you can make lasting changes that will promote a healthy lifestyle and sustainable weight loss.

How metabolism affects weight loss

Metabolism plays a crucial role in weight loss, as it refers to the body's ability to convert food into energy. A faster metabolism means that you burn calories more efficiently, making it easier to lose weight. On the other hand, a slower metabolism can make weight loss more challenging. Understanding how metabolism affects weight loss is essential for anyone looking to shed pounds and maintain a healthy lifestyle.

One way to boost metabolism naturally is by incorporating metabolism-boosting foods into your diet. Foods high in protein, such as lean meats, eggs, and legumes, can help increase your metabolism by requiring more energy to digest. Spicy foods like chili peppers can also temporarily speed up metabolism due to their thermogenic properties. Additionally, drinking green tea or coffee can increase metabolism and help burn more calories throughout the day.

In addition to eating metabolism-boosting foods, incorporating supplements into your routine can also help enhance weight loss efforts. Supplements like green tea extract, ginger, and cayenne pepper can all support a faster metabolism. However, it's essential to consult with a healthcare provider before adding any new supplements to your regimen to ensure they are safe and effective for your individual needs.

Making lifestyle changes can also have a significant impact on your metabolism and weight loss goals. Regular exercise, particularly strength training, can help increase muscle mass, which in turn boosts metabolism. Getting an adequate amount of sleep is also crucial, as sleep deprivation can slow down metabolism and lead to weight gain. Managing stress levels through activities like meditation or yoga can further support a healthy metabolism.

Finally, there are several tips and tricks you can implement to boost metabolism and aid in weight loss. Drinking plenty of water throughout the day can help keep your metabolism running efficiently. Eating smaller, more frequent meals can also prevent metabolism from slowing down. Additionally, incorporating high-intensity interval training (HIIT) into your workout routine can rev up your metabolism and burn more calories in less time. By understanding how metabolism affects weight loss and implementing these strategies, you can achieve lasting success in your weight loss journey.

Common misconceptions about metabolism

When it comes to weight loss, one of the most talked-about topics is metabolism. However, there are many misconceptions about metabolism that can lead people down the wrong path when trying to shed pounds. In this subchapter, we will address some of the most common misconceptions about metabolism and provide clarity on this important aspect of weight loss.

One common misconception about metabolism is that it is solely determined by genetics. While genetics do play a role in determining your metabolic rate, there are many lifestyle factors that can influence it as well. Factors such as diet, exercise, and sleep can all impact your metabolism and can be modified to help boost your metabolism and aid in weight loss.

Another misconception is that metabolism slows down as we age, making it harder to lose weight. While it is true that metabolism tends to slow down with age, there are ways to counteract this natural slowdown. By incorporating regular exercise and strength training into your routine, you can help maintain and even increase your metabolic rate as you age.

Many people also believe that eating less will boost their metabolism and help them lose weight faster. However, severely restricting calories can actually slow down your metabolism as your body goes into starvation mode and holds onto fat stores. It is important to fuel your body with the right amount of nutrients to keep your metabolism running efficiently.

Some people think that certain foods or supplements can magically boost their metabolism and help them shed pounds effortlessly. While there are some metabolism-boosting foods and supplements that can support weight loss, they are not a magic solution. It is important to focus on a balanced diet rich in whole foods and to incorporate regular physical activity to truly rev up your metabolism.

In conclusion, there are many misconceptions about metabolism that can hinder weight loss efforts. By understanding the true factors that influence metabolism and making lifestyle changes to support a healthy metabolism, you can achieve lasting weight loss success. It is important to focus on a holistic approach to weight loss, incorporating healthy eating habits, regular exercise, and self-care practices to boost your metabolism and reach your goals.

Chapter 2: Natural Ways to Boost Metabolism

Importance of hydration for metabolism

In order to rev up your metabolism and achieve lasting weight loss success, it is crucial to understand the importance of hydration for metabolism. Water is essential for all of the body's metabolic processes, including the breakdown of food for energy and the elimination of waste products. Dehydration can slow down your metabolism, making it harder to burn calories and lose weight. By staying properly hydrated, you can keep your metabolism running smoothly and efficiently.

One of the key ways that hydration affects metabolism is through thermogenesis, or the production of heat in the body. When you drink water, your body has to work to maintain its internal temperature, which can increase your metabolic rate. Studies have shown that drinking cold water can boost metabolism even further, as your body has to expend extra energy to warm the water to body temperature. By staying hydrated with cold water throughout the day, you can help to increase your metabolism and burn more calories.

In addition to thermogenesis, hydration is also important for the proper function of enzymes involved in metabolism. Enzymes are proteins that help to speed up chemical reactions in the body, including the breakdown of carbohydrates, fats, and proteins for energy. Without enough water, these enzymes cannot function optimally, leading to a sluggish metabolism. By drinking plenty of water throughout the day, you can support the activity of these enzymes and help to keep your metabolism in top shape.

It is important to note that not all beverages are created equal when it comes to hydration for metabolism. While water is the best choice for staying hydrated, other beverages such as coffee, tea, and soda can have a diuretic effect, leading to increased fluid loss. Alcohol can also dehydrate the body, slowing down metabolism and hindering weight loss efforts. To maximize the metabolic benefits of hydration, it is best to stick to water as your primary source of fluids throughout the day.

Overall, staying properly hydrated is essential for boosting metabolism and supporting weight loss. By drinking enough water each day, you can help to increase thermogenesis, support enzyme function, and keep your metabolism running efficiently. To optimize your metabolism even further, try adding metabolism-boosting foods and supplements to your diet, making lifestyle changes that promote a healthy metabolism, and incorporating other tips for weight loss success. With a focus on hydration and other key factors, you can rev up your metabolism and achieve lasting weight loss results.

The role of sleep in metabolism

Sleep plays a crucial role in metabolism, affecting how our bodies process and store energy from food. Lack of sleep has been linked to weight gain and obesity, as it disrupts the hormones that regulate appetite and metabolism. When we don't get enough sleep, our bodies produce more ghrelin, a hormone that stimulates hunger, and less leptin, a hormone that suppresses appetite. This can lead to increased food intake and cravings for high-calorie, sugary foods, which can sabotage weight loss efforts.

In addition to affecting appetite hormones, sleep deprivation can also impact how our bodies process carbohydrates, leading to higher blood sugar levels and insulin resistance. Insulin resistance can make it harder for the body to regulate blood sugar levels, leading to weight gain and an increased risk of developing type 2 diabetes. Getting enough sleep is essential for maintaining healthy blood sugar levels and supporting overall metabolic health.

Sleep is also important for the body's ability to repair and regenerate cells, including those involved in metabolism. During sleep, the body releases growth hormone, which plays a key role in building and repairing tissues, including muscle tissue. Adequate sleep is essential for muscle recovery and growth, which can help boost metabolism and support weight loss efforts.

Without enough sleep, the body may struggle to repair and build muscle, which can slow down metabolism and make it harder to lose weight.

Incorporating good sleep hygiene practices can help support a healthy metabolism and promote weight loss. This includes establishing a regular sleep schedule, creating a relaxing bedtime routine, and creating a comfortable sleep environment. Avoiding caffeine and electronics before bed, and practicing relaxation techniques such as meditation or deep breathing can also promote better sleep quality. Making sleep a priority can have a positive impact on metabolism and overall health.

In conclusion, sleep plays a critical role in metabolism and weight loss. Prioritizing good sleep hygiene practices and getting enough rest each night can support healthy blood sugar levels, appetite regulation, and muscle growth, all of which are essential for a well-functioning metabolism. By making sleep a priority and incorporating strategies to improve sleep quality, individuals can support their weight loss goals and improve overall metabolic health.

Incorporating stress management techniques for a healthy metabolism

Incorporating stress management techniques is crucial for maintaining a healthy metabolism. Stress can wreak havoc on our bodies, causing hormonal imbalances that can slow down our metabolism and lead to weight gain. By learning how to effectively manage stress, we can support our metabolism and promote overall well-being.

One effective stress management technique is practicing mindfulness and meditation. Taking the time to quiet the mind and focus on the present moment can help reduce stress levels and promote a sense of calm. This can have a positive impact on our metabolism, as stress hormones like cortisol are known to inhibit the body's ability to burn fat and regulate blood sugar levels.

Regular exercise is another powerful tool for managing stress and supporting a healthy metabolism. Physical activity releases endorphins, which are natural mood boosters that can help reduce stress and anxiety. Exercise also helps to regulate cortisol levels and improve insulin sensitivity, both of which are important factors in maintaining a healthy metabolism.

Incorporating relaxation techniques such as deep breathing exercises, yoga, or tai chi can also be beneficial for managing stress and supporting a healthy metabolism. These practices help to activate the body's relaxation response, which can counteract the negative effects of stress on the metabolism. By incorporating these techniques into our daily routine, we can create a more balanced and resilient body that is better equipped to handle the challenges of modern life.

Overall, by prioritizing stress management techniques in conjunction with other metabolism-boosting strategies like eating a healthy diet and getting enough sleep, we can support our body's natural ability to burn calories efficiently and maintain a healthy weight. Making these lifestyle changes can have a lasting impact on our metabolism and overall well-being, helping us to achieve lasting weight loss success.

Chapter 3: Metabolism-Boosting Foods and Supplements

Foods that can rev up your metabolism

In our quest for weight loss success, one of the key factors to consider is our metabolism. Metabolism is the process by which your body converts what you eat and drink into energy. A faster metabolism means you burn calories more efficiently, leading to weight loss. Luckily, there are certain foods that can help rev up your metabolism and aid in your weight loss journey.

One of the best metabolism-boosting foods is green tea. Green tea is rich in antioxidants called catechins, which have been shown to increase metabolism and promote fat loss. Drinking a cup of green tea daily can help kickstart your metabolism and aid in weight loss. Additionally, green tea has other health benefits such as improving brain function and reducing the risk of certain cancers.

Another metabolism-boosting food is spicy peppers. Spicy peppers contain a compound called capsaicin, which has been shown to increase metabolism and promote fat burning. Adding hot peppers to your meals can help rev up your metabolism and aid in weight loss. Additionally, spicy peppers have other health benefits such as reducing inflammation and improving heart health.

In addition to green tea and spicy peppers, protein-rich foods can also rev up your metabolism. Protein requires more energy to digest compared to carbohydrates or fats, so eating protein-rich foods can help boost your metabolism. Foods such as lean meats, fish, eggs, and legumes are all excellent sources of protein that can aid in weight loss and rev up your metabolism.

Furthermore, foods rich in fiber can also help boost your metabolism. Fiber helps to keep you feeling full and satisfied, which can prevent overeating and aid in weight loss. Foods such as fruits, vegetables, whole grains, and legumes are all excellent sources of fiber that can help rev up your metabolism and promote weight loss.

In conclusion, incorporating metabolism-boosting foods into your diet can help aid in weight loss and promote a healthier lifestyle. Green tea, spicy peppers, protein-rich foods, and fiber-rich foods are all excellent choices to rev up your metabolism and achieve lasting weight loss success. By making simple changes to your diet and lifestyle, you can boost your metabolism and achieve your weight loss goals.

The benefits of incorporating metabolism-boosting supplements

Incorporating metabolism-boosting supplements into your daily routine can have numerous benefits when it comes to weight loss and overall health. These supplements are designed to help speed up your body's metabolism, which can help you burn more calories throughout the day. By adding these supplements to your diet, you can give your metabolism the extra push it needs to help you reach your weight loss goals more efficiently.

One of the main benefits of metabolism-boosting supplements is that they can help increase your energy levels. When your metabolism is working at its optimal level, you will have more energy to tackle your daily tasks and workouts. This increased energy can help you stay motivated and focused on your weight loss journey, making it easier to stick to your healthy eating and exercise plan.

Another benefit of incorporating metabolism-boosting supplements is that they can help you burn more calories, even when you are at rest. By speeding up your metabolism, these supplements can help your body burn more calories throughout the day, which can lead to faster weight loss results. This can be especially helpful for individuals who have a slower metabolism or who struggle to lose weight despite their best efforts.

Metabolism-boosting supplements can also help improve your digestion and nutrient absorption. When your metabolism is working efficiently, your body is better able to break down the food you eat and absorb essential nutrients. This can help improve your overall health and well-being, as well as support your weight loss efforts. By incorporating these supplements into your daily routine, you can help ensure that your body is functioning at its best.

Overall, incorporating metabolism-boosting supplements into your daily routine can be a great way to support your weight loss goals and improve your overall health. These supplements can help increase your energy levels, burn more calories, improve digestion, and support nutrient absorption. By combining these supplements with a healthy diet and regular exercise, you can boost your metabolism and achieve lasting weight loss success.

How to create a balanced diet for optimal metabolism

Creating a balanced diet is crucial for optimizing your metabolism and achieving lasting weight loss success. By incorporating a variety of nutrient-dense foods into your daily meals, you can support your body's natural metabolic processes and boost your overall energy levels. Here are some tips on how to create a balanced diet that will rev up your metabolism and help you reach your weight loss goals.

First and foremost, focus on incorporating a good mix of macronutrients into your meals. This includes carbohydrates, proteins, and fats, all of which play a key role in supporting your metabolism. Carbohydrates provide your body with energy, while proteins help build and repair tissues, and fats are essential for hormone production and nutrient absorption. Aim to include a source of each macronutrient in every meal to keep your metabolism running smoothly.

In addition to macronutrients, don't forget to include plenty of micronutrients in your diet as well. Vitamins, minerals, and antioxidants are essential for supporting various metabolic processes in the body. Fruits, vegetables, whole grains, and lean proteins are all excellent sources of these important nutrients. Try to incorporate a wide variety of colorful fruits and vegetables into your meals to ensure you're getting a good mix of vitamins and minerals.

Another important aspect of creating a balanced diet for optimal metabolism is paying attention to portion sizes. Eating too much or too little can throw off your body's natural metabolic balance and hinder your weight loss efforts. Aim to eat regular, balanced meals throughout the day and listen to your body's hunger and fullness cues to determine when and how much to eat. Portion control is key to maintaining a healthy metabolism and achieving long-term weight loss success.

To further support your metabolism, consider incorporating metabolism-boosting foods and supplements into your diet. Foods like green tea, spicy peppers, and lean proteins have been shown to increase metabolic rate and promote fat burning. Additionally, supplements like caffeine, green tea extract, and L-carnitine can help enhance your body's ability to burn calories and support weight loss. Just be sure to consult with a healthcare professional before adding any new supplements to your regimen.

Lastly, don't forget to make lifestyle changes that support a healthy metabolism. Getting regular exercise, staying hydrated, managing stress, and getting enough sleep are all important factors in maintaining a balanced metabolism. By combining a nutrient-dense diet with regular physical activity and healthy lifestyle habits, you can optimize your metabolism and achieve lasting weight loss success.

Chapter 4: Metabolism-Boosting Lifestyle Changes

The impact of physical activity on metabolism

Physical activity plays a crucial role in boosting metabolism and aiding in weight loss. When we engage in physical activity, our bodies burn calories to fuel our movements. This increase in energy expenditure can help to rev up our metabolism and promote weight loss. In fact, studies have shown that regular physical activity can increase our metabolic rate, even at rest, meaning that we burn more calories throughout the day.

One of the key ways in which physical activity impacts metabolism is through the building of lean muscle mass. Muscle tissue is more metabolically active than fat tissue, meaning that the more muscle we have, the more calories we burn, even when we are not exercising. This is why strength training exercises, such as weight lifting, are so important for boosting metabolism and promoting weight loss. By incorporating strength training into our fitness routine, we can increase our muscle mass and improve our metabolic rate.

In addition to building muscle mass, physical activity can also improve insulin sensitivity, which is crucial for metabolism regulation. When we exercise, our muscles use glucose for energy, which helps to reduce blood sugar levels and improve insulin sensitivity. This can help to prevent insulin resistance, a condition that can lead to weight gain and metabolic disorders. By incorporating regular physical activity into our routine, we can help to regulate our metabolism and maintain a healthy weight.

Another way in which physical activity impacts metabolism is through the release of hormones such as endorphins and adrenaline. These hormones can help to increase our metabolic rate and promote fat burning. Additionally, physical activity can help to reduce levels of cortisol, the stress hormone, which can slow metabolism and promote weight gain. By engaging in regular physical activity, we can help to balance our hormones and support a healthy metabolism.

In conclusion, physical activity plays a crucial role in boosting metabolism and promoting weight loss. By incorporating regular exercise into our routine, we can increase our metabolic rate, build lean muscle mass, improve insulin sensitivity, and balance our hormones. Whether it's through strength training, cardio, or high-intensity interval training, finding ways to stay active can have a profound impact on our metabolism and overall health. By making physical activity a priority in our daily lives, we can support our weight loss goals and achieve lasting success.

Incorporating strength training for a faster metabolism

Incorporating strength training into your workout routine is a key component in boosting your metabolism and achieving lasting weight loss success. Strength training helps build lean muscle mass, which in turn increases your resting metabolic rate. This means that even when you are not actively working out, your body will be burning more calories throughout the day. By incorporating strength training exercises such as weight lifting, resistance bands, or bodyweight exercises into your fitness regimen, you can rev up your metabolism and achieve your weight loss goals more effectively.

In addition to building lean muscle mass, strength training can also help improve your overall body composition. As you gain muscle and lose fat, you will notice a more toned and sculpted physique. This can be incredibly motivating and rewarding as you see the physical changes in your body. By incorporating strength training into your routine, you can not only boost your metabolism but also transform your body in a positive way.

When it comes to incorporating strength training for a faster metabolism, it's important to focus on compound exercises that target multiple muscle groups at once. Exercises such as squats, deadlifts, lunges, and push-ups are great examples of compound movements that can help build strength and increase muscle mass. By incorporating these exercises into your workout routine, you can maximize the benefits of strength training and boost your metabolism even further.

In addition to incorporating strength training into your workout routine, it's also important to fuel your body with the right nutrients to support your metabolism. Protein is especially important for building and repairing muscle tissue, so be sure to include lean sources of protein such as chicken, fish, tofu, and legumes in your diet. Additionally, be sure to stay hydrated and eat a balanced diet rich in fruits, vegetables, whole grains, and healthy fats to support your overall health and metabolism.

Overall, incorporating strength training into your fitness regimen is a powerful way to boost your metabolism and achieve lasting weight loss success. By building lean muscle mass, improving your body composition, and fueling your body with the right nutrients, you can rev up your metabolism and achieve your weight loss goals more effectively. So don't be afraid to pick up those weights and start incorporating strength training into your routine today!

Ways to stay active throughout the day for a healthy metabolism

In today's fast-paced world, it can be challenging to find the time to stay active throughout the day. However, incorporating small lifestyle changes can make a big impact on your metabolism and overall health. Here are some ways to stay active throughout the day for a healthy metabolism.

One of the simplest ways to stay active is to take short breaks throughout the day to stretch and move around. This can help prevent muscle stiffness and improve circulation, both of which can boost your metabolism. Try setting a timer to remind yourself to get up and move every hour, even if it's just a quick walk around the office or a few stretches at your desk.

Another way to stay active is to incorporate exercise into your daily routine. This can be as simple as taking the stairs instead of the elevator, parking further away from your destination, or going for a walk during your lunch break. These small changes can add up over time and help keep your metabolism revved up throughout the day.

Eating metabolism-boosting foods and supplements can also help keep your energy levels up and your metabolism running smoothly. Foods like lean proteins, whole grains, fruits, and vegetables can help fuel your body and keep you feeling satisfied. Additionally, supplements like green tea extract, caffeine, and probiotics have been shown to support a healthy metabolism and aid in weight loss.

Incorporating metabolism-boosting lifestyle changes, such as getting enough sleep, managing stress, and staying hydrated, can also have a positive impact on your metabolism. Lack of sleep and high stress levels can lead to hormonal imbalances that can slow down your metabolism, so it's important to prioritize self-care and make time for relaxation and rest.

Lastly, staying active throughout the day doesn't have to be a chore. Find activities that you enjoy, whether it's going for a hike, taking a dance class, or playing a sport. The key is to find ways to move your body that feel good to you, so you're more likely to stick with them long term. By incorporating these simple strategies into your daily routine, you can boost your metabolism and set yourself up for lasting weight loss success.

Chapter 5: Metabolism-Boosting Tips for Weight Loss

Setting realistic weight loss goals based on your metabolism

When embarking on a weight loss journey, it is essential to set realistic goals based on your metabolism. Understanding your body's unique metabolic rate can help you tailor your weight loss plan to ensure long-lasting success. Metabolism plays a crucial role in how efficiently your body burns calories, so it is important to take this into consideration when setting your weight loss goals.

One way to determine your metabolism is by calculating your Basal Metabolic Rate (BMR), which is the number of calories your body needs to function at rest. This can give you a better understanding of how many calories you need to consume to maintain your current weight. From there, you can create a calorie deficit to promote weight loss. It is important to set realistic goals that are achievable based on your BMR and activity level.

Another important factor to consider when setting weight loss goals based on your metabolism is your body composition. Muscle mass plays a significant role in how efficiently your body burns calories, so incorporating strength training exercises into your routine can help boost your metabolism. Setting goals to increase muscle mass while losing fat can lead to sustainable weight loss and improved metabolic function.

In addition to exercise, focusing on metabolism-boosting foods and supplements can also help support your weight loss goals. Foods rich in protein, fiber, and healthy fats can help keep you feeling full and satisfied while also promoting a healthy metabolism. Incorporating metabolism-boosting supplements, such as green tea extract or capsaicin, can also help enhance your body's ability to burn calories.

Finally, making lifestyle changes that support a healthy metabolism can help you reach your weight loss goals more effectively. Getting an adequate amount of sleep, managing stress levels, and staying hydrated are all important factors that can influence your metabolism. By incorporating these lifestyle changes into your weight loss plan, you can create a sustainable and effective approach to achieving your goals. Remember, setting realistic goals based on your metabolism is key to long-term weight loss success.

Tracking progress and adjusting your plan accordingly

Tracking progress is an essential component of any successful weight loss journey. By keeping track of your food intake, exercise regimen, and overall progress, you can identify patterns, setbacks, and areas for improvement. One of the most effective ways to track your progress is by keeping a food journal. Write down everything you eat and drink throughout the day, along with the portion sizes and any relevant nutritional information. This will help you identify any unhealthy eating habits and make necessary adjustments to your diet.

In addition to tracking your food intake, it's also important to monitor your exercise routine and overall physical activity. Keeping a workout log can help you stay accountable and motivated, while also allowing you to track your progress over time. Whether you prefer cardio, strength training, or a combination of both, make sure to record the type of exercise, duration, and intensity to ensure you are consistently challenging yourself and making progress towards your weight loss goals.

As you track your progress, it's important to be flexible and willing to adjust your plan accordingly. Weight loss is not a linear process, and there will inevitably be ups and downs along the way. If you hit a plateau or experience setbacks, don't get discouraged. Instead, use this as an opportunity to reassess your plan, identify potential obstacles, and make necessary adjustments. This might involve changing up your exercise routine, trying new metabolism-boosting foods and supplements, or seeking support from a weight loss coach or support group.

In addition to tracking your progress and adjusting your plan accordingly, it's also important to focus on making sustainable lifestyle changes that will support your long-term weight loss success. This includes prioritizing sleep, managing stress, and practicing mindfulness. By prioritizing self-care and overall well-being, you can create a solid foundation for lasting weight loss success and improved metabolism. Remember, weight loss is not just about the numbers on the scale, but also about feeling healthier, happier, and more confident in your own skin.

In conclusion, tracking progress and adjusting your plan accordingly are essential components of any successful weight loss journey. By keeping a food journal, monitoring your exercise routine, and being flexible and open to making necessary adjustments, you can stay on track towards your weight loss goals. Additionally, focusing on sustainable lifestyle changes, such as prioritizing sleep, managing stress, and practicing mindfulness, can support your long-term success and overall well-being. Remember, weight loss is a journey, not a destination, so be patient, stay committed, and celebrate your progress along the way.

Staying motivated and consistent with your metabolism-boosting lifestyle changes

Staying motivated and consistent with your metabolism-boosting lifestyle changes is crucial for long-term success in achieving and maintaining weight loss goals. It can be challenging to make lasting changes to your diet and exercise routine, but with the right mindset and strategies, you can stay on track and see results. Here are some tips to help you stay motivated and consistent on your journey to rev up your metabolism and achieve lasting weight loss success.

One key to staying motivated is to set realistic and achievable goals for yourself. Instead of focusing on a specific number on the scale, aim to make small, sustainable changes to your lifestyle that will support a healthy metabolism. For example, you could set a goal to add more metabolism-boosting foods to your diet each week or to incorporate a new workout routine into your schedule. By setting achievable goals, you can track your progress and celebrate your successes along the way.

Another important aspect of staying motivated is to find support from others who share your goals. Whether you join a weight loss support group, work with a personal trainer, or enlist the help of a friend or family member, having someone to encourage and hold you accountable can make a big difference in staying consistent with your lifestyle changes. Surround yourself with positive influences who will support your efforts and cheer you on as you work towards your goals.

In addition to setting goals and finding support, it's important to stay mindful of your progress and celebrate your achievements along the way. Keep a journal to track your daily habits and note any changes you see in your energy levels, mood, or weight. Celebrate small victories, such as choosing a healthy snack over a sugary treat or completing a challenging workout, to stay motivated and focused on your long-term goals.

To stay consistent with your metabolism-boosting lifestyle changes, it's also important to prioritize self-care and make time for activities that help reduce stress and promote overall well-being. Getting enough sleep, practicing relaxation techniques like yoga or meditation, and finding ways to unwind and relax can all support a healthy metabolism and help you stay motivated on your weight loss journey.

By setting realistic goals, finding support, tracking your progress, celebrating your achievements, and prioritizing self-care, you can stay motivated and consistent with your metabolism-boosting lifestyle changes. With dedication and perseverance, you can achieve lasting weight loss success and enjoy a healthier, more energetic life. Remember that change takes time and effort, but with the right mindset and strategies, you can rev up your metabolism and achieve your weight loss goals for good.

23

Chapter 6: Maintaining a Healthy Metabolism for Lasting Weight Loss Success

Strategies for long-term weight maintenance

In this subchapter, we will explore strategies for long-term weight maintenance to help you achieve lasting success in your weight loss journey. These strategies are designed to support your metabolism, promote healthy habits, and prevent weight regain in the future. By implementing these tips and making them a part of your daily routine, you can ensure that you not only reach your weight loss goals but also maintain them for the long term.

One of the key strategies for long-term weight maintenance is to focus on natural ways to boost your metabolism. This includes incorporating physical activity into your daily routine, such as regular exercise, strength training, and cardiovascular workouts. By staying active and moving your body regularly, you can keep your metabolism revved up and burning calories efficiently. Additionally, getting enough sleep, managing stress levels, and staying hydrated are all important factors that can help support a healthy metabolism and prevent weight gain in the future.

Another important aspect of maintaining weight loss is to focus on metabolism-boosting foods and supplements. Incorporating nutrient-dense foods into your diet, such as fruits, vegetables, lean proteins, and whole grains, can help support a healthy metabolism and provide your body with the energy it needs to function optimally. Additionally, certain supplements, such as green tea extract, caffeine, and protein powders, can help boost your metabolism and support weight loss efforts. However, it's important to consult with a healthcare professional before starting any new supplements to ensure they are safe and effective for you.

Making metabolism-boosting lifestyle changes is also crucial for long-term weight maintenance. This includes creating a supportive environment at home and work, setting realistic goals, and finding ways to stay motivated and accountable. Surrounding yourself with supportive friends and family, creating a meal plan, and tracking your progress can all help you stay on track and prevent weight regain in the future. Additionally, finding healthy ways to cope with stress, managing your time effectively, and practicing mindful eating can all contribute to long-term weight maintenance and overall well-being.

Finally, incorporating metabolism-boosting tips for weight loss into your daily routine can help you achieve lasting success. This includes eating smaller, more frequent meals throughout the day, staying hydrated, and incorporating high-intensity interval training (HIIT) into your workout routine. Additionally, practicing portion control, avoiding processed foods, and finding ways to stay active throughout the day, such as taking the stairs or going for a walk, can all help support a healthy metabolism and prevent weight regain in the future. By implementing these strategies and making them a part of your daily routine, you can achieve lasting weight loss success and maintain a healthy weight for the long term.

The importance of regular check-ins and adjustments to your metabolism-boosting plan

In order to achieve lasting weight loss success, it is crucial to regularly check in and make adjustments to your metabolism-boosting plan. Your metabolism is not a static entity; it can fluctuate based on a variety of factors such as age, activity level, and overall health. By staying proactive and monitoring your progress, you can ensure that your metabolism-boosting efforts are still effective and making a positive impact on your weight loss goals.

One of the key reasons why regular check-ins are important is to assess whether your current plan is still working for you. As your body adapts to changes in diet and exercise, it may become more efficient at burning calories and storing fat. By checking in regularly, you can identify any plateaus or setbacks and make the necessary adjustments to keep your metabolism revved up and your weight loss on track.

Another important aspect of regular check-ins is to hold yourself accountable and stay motivated. It can be easy to fall off track or lose sight of your goals if you are not actively monitoring your progress. By scheduling regular check-ins with yourself or a support system, you can stay accountable to your metabolism-boosting plan and stay motivated to continue making healthy choices.

In addition to regular check-ins, it is also important to make adjustments to your metabolism-boosting plan as needed. This could include increasing the intensity of your workouts, trying new metabolism-boosting foods or supplements, or incorporating new lifestyle changes that support a healthy metabolism. By staying flexible and open to making adjustments, you can ensure that your metabolism stays revved up and continues to support your weight loss goals.

Overall, regular check-ins and adjustments are essential for maintaining a metabolism-boosting plan that is effective and sustainable in the long term. By staying proactive, accountable, and willing to make changes as needed, you can ensure that your metabolism is working for you and not against you in your weight loss journey. So, be sure to schedule regular check-ins and be open to making adjustments as needed to keep your metabolism revved up and your weight loss goals on track.

Celebrating your successes and staying committed to a healthy lifestyle

Celebrating your successes is an important part of staying committed to a healthy lifestyle. When you reach a weight loss goal or make a positive change in your diet or exercise routine, it's important to take the time to acknowledge and celebrate your achievements. This can help to reinforce your commitment to your goals and motivate you to continue making healthy choices.

One way to celebrate your successes is to treat yourself to something special, such as a massage, a new workout outfit, or a healthy meal at your favorite restaurant. You could also celebrate by sharing your achievements with friends and family, who can offer support and encouragement as you continue on your weight loss journey. Taking the time to celebrate your successes can help you to stay motivated and focused on your goals.

In addition to celebrating your successes, it's important to stay committed to a healthy lifestyle in order to maintain your weight loss and continue to see results. This means making sustainable changes to your diet and exercise routine that you can stick to in the long term. For example, instead of following a fad diet or extreme exercise plan, focus on making small, manageable changes that you can maintain over time.

One way to stay committed to a healthy lifestyle is to incorporate metabolism-boosting foods and supplements into your diet. These foods and supplements can help to increase your metabolism, making it easier to burn calories and lose weight. Some examples of metabolism-boosting foods include lean proteins, whole grains, fruits, and vegetables, while supplements like green tea extract and caffeine can also help to boost your metabolism.

Finally, it's important to remember that staying committed to a healthy lifestyle is a journey, not a destination. There will be ups and downs along the way, but by celebrating your successes, making sustainable changes to your diet and exercise routine, and incorporating metabolism-boosting foods and supplements into your daily routine, you can achieve lasting weight loss success. By staying committed and focused on your goals, you can create a healthier, happier life for yourself.

www.ingramcontent.com/pod-product-compliance
Lightning Source LLC
Chambersburg PA
CBHW072345270726
48659CB00023B/2399